Table of Contents

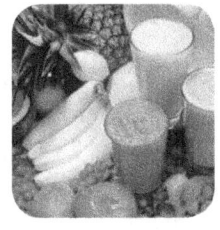 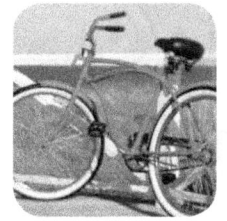 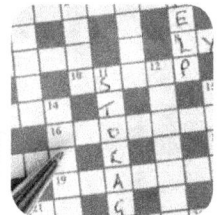

Introduction

The news is full of stories about ways to stay healthy, eat right, and keep fit. Along with keeping their bodies healthy, people want to keep their minds sharp as they age. They also want to avoid brain disorders such as Alzheimer's disease.

Currently, Alzheimer's disease has no known cure, but recent research results are raising hopes that someday it might be possible to delay, slow down, or even prevent this devastating disease. The National Institute on Aging (NIA), part of the National Institutes of Health (NIH) at the U.S. Department of Health and Human Services, is the lead Federal agency for research related to Alzheimer's disease, mild cognitive impairment (MCI), and age-related cognitive decline. This booklet summarizes what scientists have learned so far and where research is headed.

There is no definitive evidence yet about what can prevent Alzheimer's or age-related cognitive decline. What we do know is that a healthy lifestyle—one that includes a healthy diet, physical activity, appropriate weight, and no smoking—can maintain and improve overall health and well-being. Making healthy choices can also lower the risk of certain chronic diseases, like heart disease and diabetes, and scientists are very interested in the possibility that a healthy lifestyle might have a beneficial effect on Alzheimer's as well. In the meantime, as research continues to pinpoint what works to prevent Alzheimer's, people of all ages can benefit from taking positive steps to get and stay healthy. (See "So, What Can You Do?" page 21.)

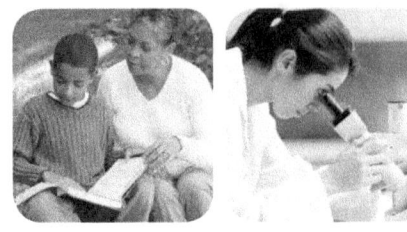 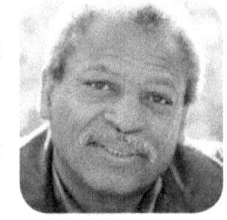

What Is Alzheimer's Disease?

Alzheimer's is an age-related brain disease that gradually destroys a person's memory and thinking skills and, eventually, even the ability to carry out the simplest tasks. Alzheimer's is the most common cause of dementia, a loss of cognitive functioning and behavioral abilities so severe that it interferes with a person's daily life and activities.

Some mild forgetfulness is normal as people get older. But sometimes memory or other thinking problems are serious—they make it hard to do everyday things like driving, shopping, 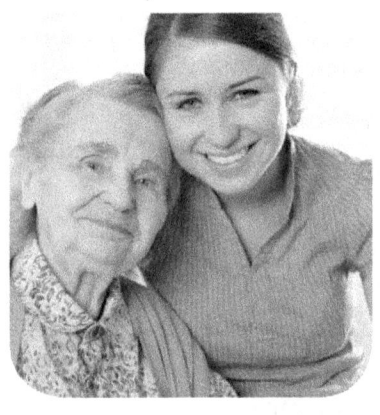 or even talking with a friend. For example, people with MCI have memory or other thinking problems greater than normal for their age and education but can still function independently. MCI often, but not always, leads to Alzheimer's dementia. Research is helping scientists better understand cognitive changes related to aging.

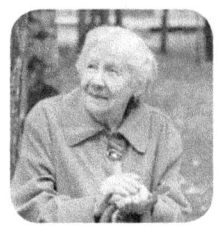 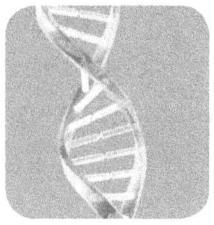 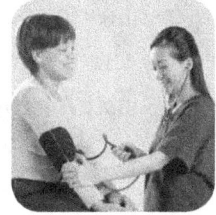

Risk Factors for Alzheimer's Disease

Alzheimer's is a complex disease that progresses over many years, like diabetes, heart disease, and other chronic conditions. A number of factors may increase or decrease a person's chances of developing the disease. These risk factors include age, genetics, environment, and lifestyle. The importance of these factors may be different for different people. Some risk factors can be changed or controlled while others cannot.

Research shows that Alzheimer's disease causes changes in the brain years and even decades before the first symptoms appear, so even people who seem free of the disease today may be at risk. Scientists are developing sophisticated tests to help identify who is most likely to develop symptoms of Alzheimer's. Ultimately, they hope to prevent or delay dementia in these high-risk individuals. (See "Finding Out Who Is At Risk," page 20.)

Age

Age is the best known risk factor for Alzheimer's disease. The risk of developing the disease doubles every 5 years after age 65. Alzheimer's becomes increasingly common as people reach their 80s, 90s, and beyond. These facts are significant because the number of older adults is growing. The U.S. Census Bureau estimates that Americans 65 and older will grow from

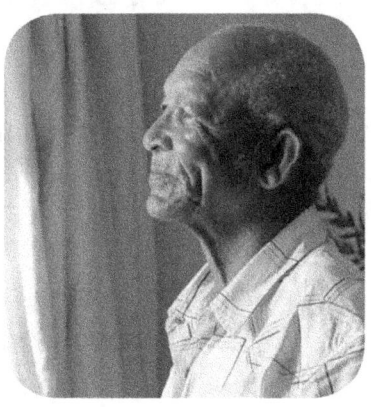

13 percent of the population today to nearly 20 percent in 2030. The group with the highest risk of Alzheimer's—those older than 85—is the fastest growing age group.

Genetics

The more researchers learn about Alzheimer's disease, the more they realize that genes play an important role in its development. Scientists have found genetic links to both early-onset and late-onset Alzheimer's disease.

Early-onset Alzheimer's is rare, accounting for only about 5 percent of people with the disease. Its symptoms usually appear when people are in their 30s, 40s, and 50s. Most cases of early-onset Alzheimer's are familial, caused by mutations (permanent changes) in one of three known genes inherited from a parent.

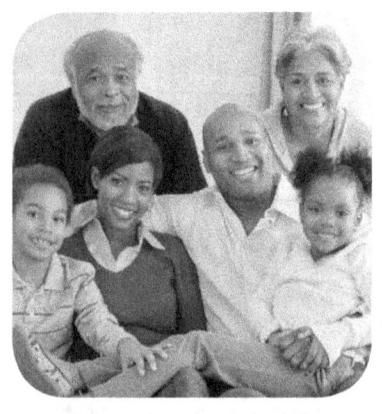

Late-onset Alzheimer's disease, the most common type, typically becomes evident after age 60. The causes of late-onset Alzheimer's are not yet completely understood, but researchers have identified several risk-factor genes. One of those genes, called apolipoprotein E (APOE), has three forms, or alleles (ε2, ε3, and ε4). One form, APOE ε4, increases a person's risk of getting the disease. It is present in about 25 to 30 percent of the population. However, carrying APOE ε4 does not necessarily mean that a person will develop Alzheimer's, and people without APOE ε4 can develop the disease.

Scientists have identified a number of other genes that may increase a person's risk for late-onset Alzheimer's. More studies are needed to assess the role these genes may play and to search for additional risk-factor genes. Knowing about these genes can help researchers more effectively test possible treatments and prevention strategies in people who are at risk of developing Alzheimer's—ideally, before symptoms appear.

Genetic testing cannot predict who will or will not develop late-onset Alzheimer's. Currently, it is used only in research settings and for people with a family history of early-onset Alzheimer's disease. This type of testing is not recommended for people at risk of late-onset Alzheimer's. It is not conclusive, and its primary value at this point remains in research settings.

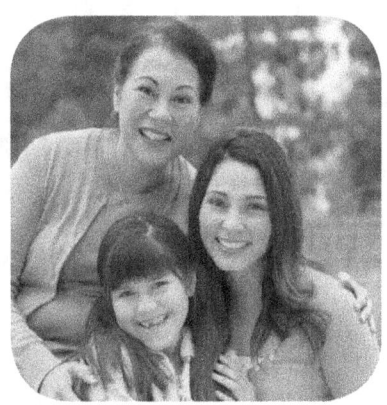

To Learn More

The NIA's Alzheimer's Disease Education and Referral (ADEAR) Center answers questions and provides free publications about Alzheimer's disease and other types of dementia. To learn more about genetics, see the "Alzheimer's Disease Genetics Fact Sheet," *www.nia.nih.gov/alzheimers/publication/alzheimers-disease-genetics-fact-sheet.*

Understanding Scientific Findings in the News

Results of medical research studies appear in the headlines every day, raising and dashing hopes that cures for devastating diseases are right around the corner. It can be hard to know what to think about these study findings. Knowing the type of study and how it was conducted can help put the results into perspective.

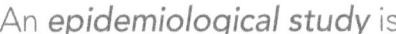

An *epidemiological study* is an observational study that looks for common factors that might explain why or how a disease occurs in a certain group of people. Scientists gather information about people who are going about their daily lives, then analyze the data to see which behaviors or environmental factors are linked to a disease or other outcome.

Epidemiological studies can't tell us for sure that these factors actually cause or prevent the disease or health condition. Based on epidemiological studies of Alzheimer's disease, scientists can report that a finding is or is not "associated with" Alzheimer's, not whether it directly affects development or progression of the disease.

For example, some epidemiological studies have found that people who exercise are less likely than inactive people to develop Alzheimer's disease. But, people who exercise tend to be healthier in other ways than those who do not exercise, such as having lower rates of heart disease or eating a nutritious diet. We don't know if their lower Alzheimer's risk results from exercise, healthier eating, reduced risk of other diseases, a combination of those factors, or something else. So, we don't know if exercising—including how much and how often—will directly lower Alzheimer's risk.

Scientists also use *in vitro (test tube) studies* and *animal studies* to learn about disease. These types of studies control specific factors that might influence a research result. This approach allows researchers to be more certain about possible causes of a disease. However, showing a cause-and-effect relationship in tissue samples or animals does not mean that the relationship will be the same in humans.

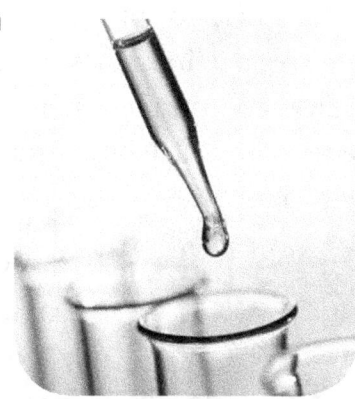

Randomized clinical trials are the best way to test directly in people the safety, effectiveness, and side effects of a medication or other treatment. In this type of research, some participants are randomly assigned to receive the intervention being tested—say, medication or exercise—while others receive a placebo (such as an inactive pill or a control intervention). Any differences in outcome between the groups should result from the treatment rather than other differences between the participants.

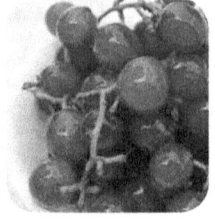 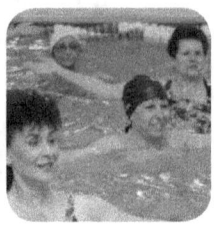 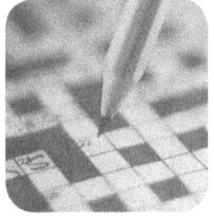

The Search for Alzheimer's Prevention Strategies

Unlike age and genetics, certain health and lifestyle factors associated with Alzheimer's disease risk may be controlled. Scientists are exploring prevention strategies to determine whether or not things like exercise, diet, and "brain games" can help delay or prevent Alzheimer's disease and age-related cognitive decline. They are also investigating how certain medical conditions, such as high cholesterol, high blood pressure, and diabetes, influence risk for cognitive impairment.

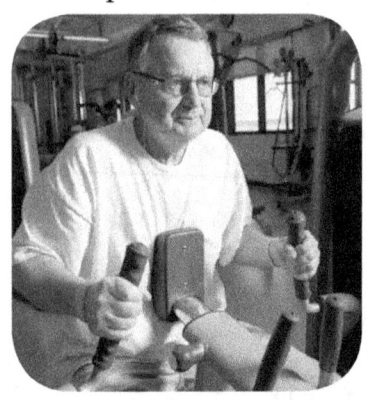

So far, studies have not demonstrated that, over the long term, health or lifestyle factors can prevent or slow Alzheimer's disease or age-related cognitive decline. Similarly, clinical trial results do not support the use of any particular medication or dietary supplement to prevent these conditions.

Promising research in these areas is underway. The NIA supports more than 30 clinical trials, including many that are investigating possible ways to prevent or delay Alzheimer's disease or age-related cognitive decline. Observational studies have *associated* factors such as physical activity, blood pressure, and diabetes control with changes in risk. More research is needed to determine whether these factors can in fact directly help prevent Alzheimer's or cognitive decline.

Do Exercise and Physical Activity Protect the Brain?

Exercise and other types of physical activity have many benefits. Studies show that they are good for our hearts, waistlines, and ability to carry out everyday activities. Epidemiological studies and some intervention studies suggest that physical exercise may also play a role in reducing risk for Alzheimer's disease and age-related cognitive decline.

Animal studies point to why this might be so. Exercise increases both the number of small blood vessels that supply blood to the brain and the number of connections between nerve cells in older rats and mice. In addition, researchers have found that exercise raises the level of a nerve growth factor (a protein key to brain health) in an area of the brain that is important to memory and learning.

Researchers have also shown that exercise can stimulate the human brain's ability to maintain old network connections and make new ones that are vital to healthy cognition. In a year-long study, 65 older people exercised daily, doing either an aerobic exercise program of walking for 40 minutes or a nonaerobic program of stretching and toning exercises. At the end of the trial, the walking group showed improved connectivity in the part of the brain engaged in daydreaming, envisioning the future, and recalling the past. The walking group also improved on executive function, the ability to plan and organize tasks such as cooking a meal.

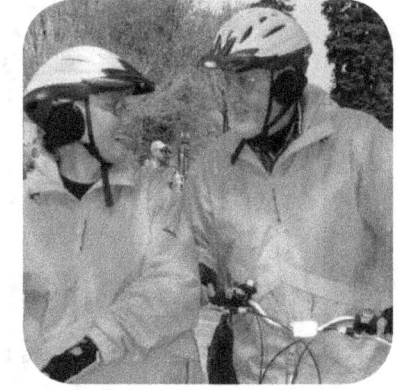

Several other clinical trials are exploring further the effect of physical activity on the risk of Alzheimer's and cognitive decline. Other NIA-supported research is examining whether exercise can delay the development of Alzheimer's disease in people with MCI. Findings from these and other clinical trials will show more definitively whether exercise helps protect our brains from cognitive impairment.

Does Diet Matter?

A number of studies suggest that eating certain foods may help keep the brain healthy—and that others can be detrimental to 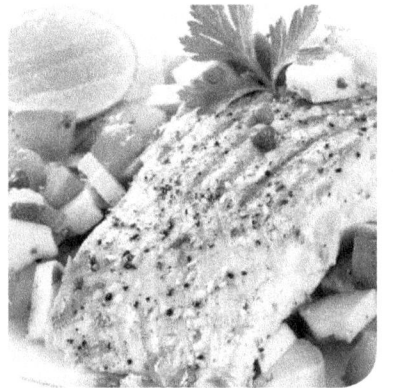 cognitive health. A diet that includes lots of fruits, vegetables, and whole grains and is low in fat and added sugar can reduce the risk of many chronic diseases, including heart disease and type 2 diabetes. Researchers are looking at whether a healthy diet also can help preserve cognitive function or reduce the risk of Alzheimer's.

Studies have found, for example, that a diet rich in vegetables, especially green leafy vegetables and cruciferous vegetables like broccoli, is associated with a reduced rate of cognitive decline. One epidemiological study reported that people who ate a "Mediterranean diet" had a 28 percent lower risk of developing MCI and a 48 percent lower risk of progressing from MCI to Alzheimer's disease. A Mediterranean diet includes vegetables, legumes, fruits, cereals, fish, olive oil, mild to moderate amounts of alcohol, and low amounts of saturated fats, dairy products, meat, and poultry.

While some foods may stave off cognitive decline, other foods, such as saturated fats and refined carbohydrates (white sugar, for example), may pose a problem. In one study, scientists fed rats a "Western" diet high in fats and simple carbohydrates for 90 days. The results: rats fed this high-energy diet performed significantly worse on certain memory tests than rats fed a diet containing one-third the fat. Notably, the rats scored poorly on tests that involve the hippocampus, a part of the brain that plays a major role in learning and memory.

Some scientists have focused on DHA (docosahexaenoic acid), an omega-3 fatty acid found in salmon and certain other fish. Studies in mice specially bred to have features of Alzheimer's disease found that DHA reduces beta-amyloid plaques, abnormal protein deposits in the brain that are a hallmark of Alzheimer's. Although a clinical trial of DHA showed no impact on people with mild to moderate Alzheimer's disease, it is possible that DHA supplements could be effective if started before cognitive symptoms appear.

These findings are of great interest and suggest possible areas for future study. The NIA supports clinical trials to examine the relationship between several dietary components and Alzheimer's disease and cognitive decline.

What Is the Effect of Other Chronic Diseases?

Age-related diseases and conditions—such as vascular disease, high blood pressure, heart disease, and type 2 diabetes—may increase the risk of Alzheimer's and cognitive decline. Many studies are looking at whether this risk can be reduced by preventing or controlling these diseases and conditions through medication or changes in diet and exercise.

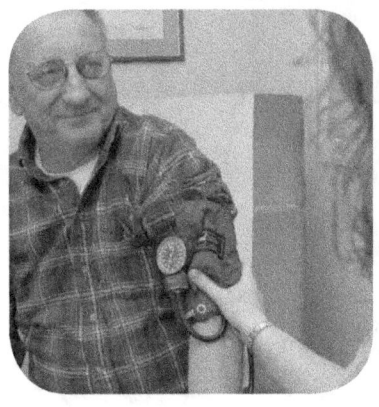

Much of the evidence about possible ties between vascular diseases and Alzheimer's risk comes from observational studies. For example, high cholesterol levels and obesity during midlife—known risk factors for heart disease—have also been linked to increased risk of Alzheimer's disease. High blood pressure may be another risk factor.

What About Vitamins and Dietary Supplements?

Can any vitamins or dietary supplements protect the brain from Alzheimer's disease and cognitive decline? One area of research focuses on *antioxidants*, natural substances that appear to fight damage caused by molecules called free radicals. Other studies are looking at a compound called resveratrol.

As a person ages, free radicals can build up in nerve cells, causing damage that might contribute to Alzheimer's. Some epidemiological and laboratory studies suggest that antioxidants from food or dietary supplements help prevent this oxidative damage—and lower the risk of Alzheimer's disease—but other studies have shown no effect. Vitamin E, vitamin C, B vitamins, ginkgo biloba, and coenzyme Q have all been tested in clinical trials, but none has proven effective in preventing or slowing down Alzheimer's disease.

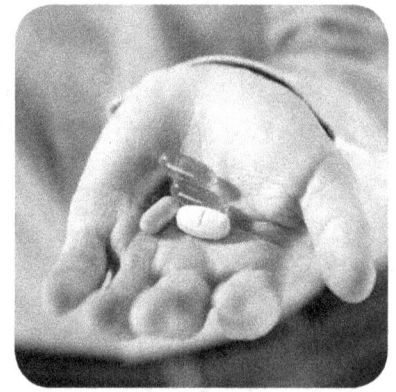

Resveratrol, a compound found in red grapes as well as supplements, appears to have properties that may help protect the brain. Observational studies have shown that moderate consumption of red wine is associated with a lower incidence of Alzheimer's disease, and animal studies have shown that resveratrol can reduce beta-amyloid deposits in the brain. Resveratrol also appears to affect the biological processes of aging-related diseases, including Alzheimer's. An NIA-supported clinical trial will test the effects of resveratrol in people with Alzheimer's disease.

One NIH clinical trial is looking at how lowering blood pressure to or below current recommended levels may affect cognitive decline and the development of MCI and Alzheimer's disease. Participants are older adults with high systolic blood pressure who have a history of heart disease or stroke, or are at risk for those conditions.

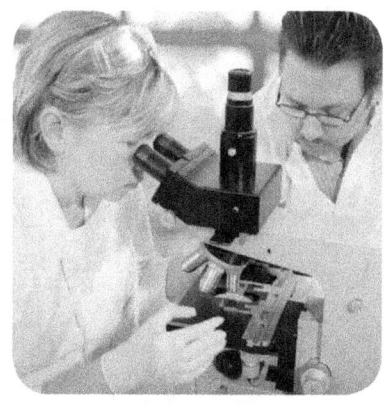

Diabetes is another disease that has been linked to Alzheimer's. Previous research suggests that abnormal insulin production (insulin is the hormone involved in diabetes) contributes to Alzheimer's-related brain changes. Can restoring normal insulin function in the brain provide cognitive benefits?

The results so far are mixed. One large NIH-funded clinical trial compared intensive glucose-lowering treatment with standard treatment in nearly 3,000 older adults with diabetes. After 40 months, the two groups showed no significant difference in cognitive function. But pilot testing of an insulin nasal spray has shown promising results. A clinical trial is testing this potential treatment in older adults with MCI or mild to moderate Alzheimer's disease to see if it can improve memory and daily functioning.

Additional studies and clinical trials are looking at cardiovascular and diabetes medications to see if they might prevent Alzheimer's disease. These therapies include aspirin, medications used to treat high blood pressure and other heart conditions, and the diabetes drugs metformin and pioglitazone.

Is Keeping Your Brain Active Important?

Staying cognitively active throughout life—via social engagement or intellectual stimulation—is associated with a lower

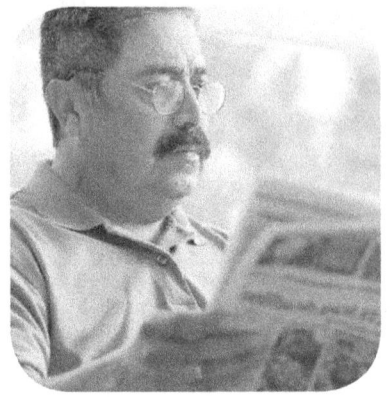

risk of Alzheimer's disease. Several observational studies link continued cognitive health with social engagement through work, volunteering, or living with someone. Mentally stimulating activities such as reading books and magazines, going to lectures, and playing games are also linked to keeping the mind sharp.

In a large study of healthy older people, researchers found a relationship between more frequent social activity and better cognitive function. It is not clear whether improved cognition resulted from the social interaction itself or from related factors, such as increased intellectual stimulation, that generally accompany social interaction. Other studies are exploring these relationships.

Intellectually stimulating activities may also reduce the risk of Alzheimer's, studies show. One large observational study looked at the impact of ordinary activities like listening to the radio, reading newspapers, playing puzzle games, and visiting

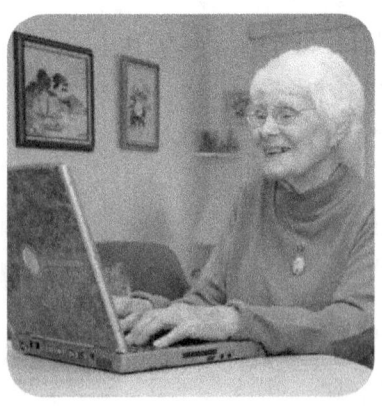

museums. Investigators asked more than 700 older nuns, priests, and religious brothers to describe the amount of time they spent doing these activities. After 4 years, the risk of developing Alzheimer's disease was 47 percent lower, on average, for those who did the activities most often than for those who did them least frequently.

How Might an Active Brain Prevent Alzheimer's?

The reasons for the apparent link between social engagement or intellectual stimulation and Alzheimer's risk aren't entirely clear, but scientists offer these possibilities:

- Such activities may protect the brain by establishing "cognitive reserve," the brain's ability to operate effectively even when it is damaged or some brain function is disrupted.

- These activities may help the brain become more adaptable in some mental functions, so it can compensate for declines in other functions.

- People who engage in these activities may have other lifestyle factors that protect them against Alzheimer's disease.

- Less engagement with other people or in intellectually stimulating activities could be the result of very early effects of Alzheimer's rather than its cause.

A more recent study showed that people with less education who engaged in activities like reading, doing crossword puzzles, and writing letters performed as well on memory tests as their better-educated peers. Having fewer years of education has been associated with a higher risk of dementia. More research is needed to see if everyday cognitive activities can reduce the risk of cognitive decline in people with less education.

Formal cognitive training also seems to have cognitive benefits. In the Advanced Cognitive Training for Independent and Vital Elderly (ACTIVE) trial, for example, healthy adults 65 and older participated in 10 sessions of memory training, reasoning training, or processing-speed training. The sessions improved participants' mental skills in the area in which they were trained. These improvements persisted 10 years after the training was complete.

Another approach is testing the impact of formal cognitive training, with and without aerobic exercise. For example, an NIA-funded clinical trial is investigating the effectiveness of cognitive training, alone and combined with aerobic exercise, in people with MCI to see if it can prevent or delay Alzheimer's disease. Other trials are underway in healthy older adults to see if exercise and/or cognitive training (for example, a demanding video game) can delay or prevent age-related cognitive decline.

Other types of formal cognitive training are being studied in healthy older adults to explore their impact on age-related cognitive decline. Types of training being tested in NIA-funded trials include learning digital photography or quilting and volunteering at local schools.

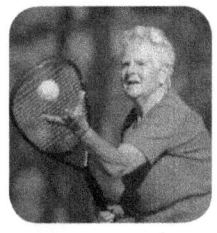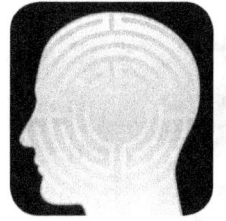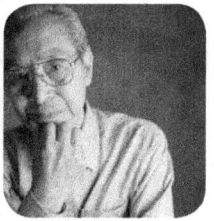

Other Clues to Alzheimer's Prevention

The quest for ways to prevent Alzheimer's disease is part of a broad research program that is exploring a number of possibilities. For example, scientists are looking at caregiver stress and physical frailty as possible risk factors for Alzheimer's disease and MCI. Other areas of interest include hormones and immunization.

Hormones

Scientists are studying hormones—especially those taken by older women as menopausal hormone therapy—for their potential ability to prevent or delay Alzheimer's disease and age-related cognitive decline. Several clinical trials are testing forms of estrogen as well as testosterone and other hormones in both healthy older adults and those with MCI.

Hormones such as estrogen and progesterone have important effects on the brain, many of which could relate to cognitive aging and Alzheimer's disease. Over the years, research has led to conflicting reports as to whether menopausal hormone therapy can prevent cognitive decline in postmenopausal women.

Some animal and observational studies comparing women who did and did not take estrogen have shown that the hormone may benefit cognition. However, clinical trials of estrogen and progestin in older women have generally failed to show similar beneficial effects. In fact, one large study showed that prolonged treatment with these hormones actually increased the risk of dementia in women 65 and older.

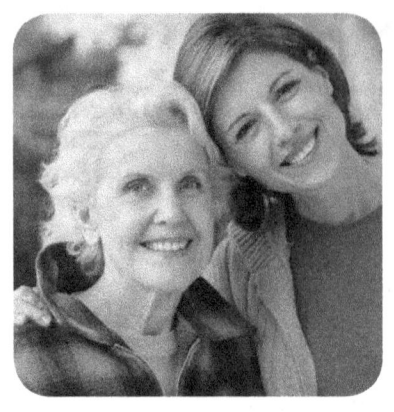

Researchers now wonder if it may be better for women to start taking hormones closer to menopause. NIA-funded clinical trials are studying the timing of menopausal hormone therapy on cognition and other health factors.

Other hormones being studied in clinical trials for their effects on Alzheimer's and cognitive decline include testosterone, which is being tested in older men with MCI and low levels of the hormone; growth hormone releasing hormone (GHRH), in healthy older adults and those with early MCI; and DHEA, in healthy postmenopausal women.

Immunization

The idea of a vaccine to prevent Alzheimer's disease is under scrutiny as well. Early vaccine studies in mice were so successful in reducing deposits of Alzheimer's-related proteins in the brain and improving performance on memory tests that investigators conducted preliminary clinical trials in humans with Alzheimer's disease. These studies had to be stopped, however, because life-threatening brain inflammation occurred in some participants.

Scientists continue to refine this approach, hoping to maintain the vaccine's possible benefits while reducing side effects. Several pharmaceutical companies are testing potential vaccines for safety and effectiveness in clinical trials.

The NIA is also supporting a clinical trial testing whether intravenous immunoglobulin (IVIg), a blood product containing naturally occurring antibodies that is used to treat immune-system disorders, may improve cognition by clearing Alzheimer's plaques from the brain.

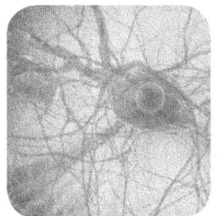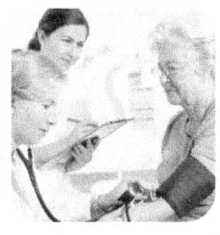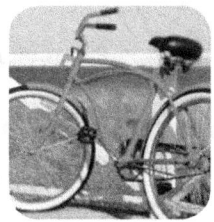

The Path to Developing New Treatments

Clinical trials will ultimately tell us what prevents or delays Alzheimer's and cognitive decline. But other areas of research are critical for developing successful prevention strategies. Basic studies of the cellular and molecular roots of Alzheimer's are revealing a wide range of processes that interfere with, or enhance, the function and survival of nerve cells in the brain. These basic research discoveries point to new targets for Alzheimer's treatment.

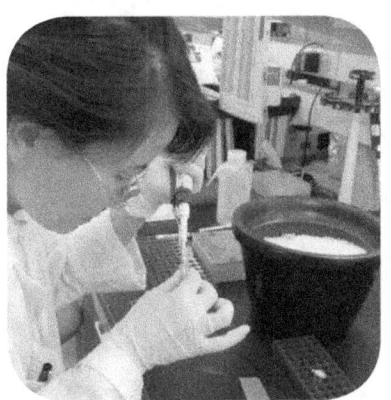

Translational studies build on the findings from basic research to develop new drugs and interventions. More than 60 projects in the NIA's translational research portfolio have supported early drug discovery and early clinical development of new treatment compounds for Alzheimer's. The goal is to expand possible avenues for Alzheimer's prevention and treatment and, eventually, to increase the number of therapies that can be tested in humans.

Finding Out Who Is At Risk

Several clinical trials of medications and other therapies have failed to improve memory and other thinking skills in people diagnosed with Alzheimer's disease. Scientists want to try some of these interventions earlier in the disease process, in cognitively normal people at high risk of developing Alzheimer's, to see if they can prevent or delay the onset of the disease.

To conduct such studies, researchers must first figure out which people without Alzheimer's symptoms are in fact at risk of developing the disease. Because the brain damage caused by Alzheimer's begins years before memory loss and other symptoms may appear, scientists are developing methods to detect biological changes related to Alzheimer's disease at its earliest stages.

Researchers are finding that changes in certain proteins in blood and cerebrospinal fluid and results of brain scans can indicate early Alzheimer's-like changes in the brain. Understanding more about these "biomarkers" may reveal how Alzheimer's disease begins and develops. Biomarkers also may help scientists track whether certain medications have their intended effects early in the course of the disease.

An NIA-led public-private partnership—the Alzheimer's Disease Neuroimaging Initiative (ADNI)—is examining the relationship between these biomarkers and cognitive changes in older participants who are cognitively normal or have MCI or Alzheimer's. Scientists hope the results will help identify ways to determine the risk of Alzheimer's disease more accurately in people without dementia symptoms.

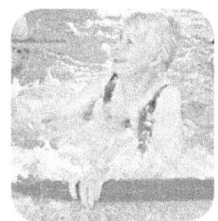 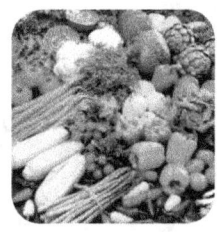 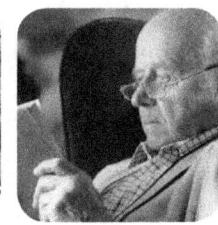

So, What Can You Do?

You can do many things that may keep your brain healthy and your body fit—and help scientists find ways to prevent Alzheimer's.

Stay Healthy

Many actions lower the risk of chronic diseases and boost overall health and well-being. As we learn more about the role they may play in Alzheimer's disease risk, health experts encourage all adults to:

- exercise regularly
- eat a healthy diet rich in fruits and vegetables
- engage in social and intellectually stimulating activities
- control type 2 diabetes
- lower high blood pressure levels
- lower high blood cholesterol levels
- maintain a healthy weight
- stop smoking
- get treatment for depression

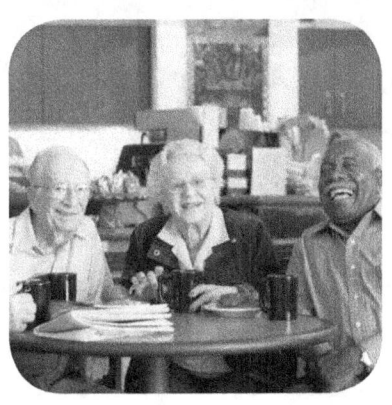

Scientists do not yet know if these healthy habits can directly prevent or delay Alzheimer's disease or age-related cognitive decline. As research continues, it's important to note the many benefits these habits have for overall health and well-being.

Participate in Research

Whether or not you have signs of Alzheimer's, you can take one more important action—volunteer to participate in clinical trials and studies. Volunteers want to make a valuable contribution that will help scientists, people with Alzheimer's, and their families. People who participate in this kind of research also have regular contact with medical experts who have lots of experience and a broad perspective on the disease.

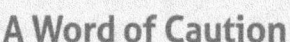

To learn more about clinical trials or to find study sites near you, contact the NIA's Alzheimer's Disease Education and Referral (ADEAR) Center at 1-800-438-4380 or visit *www.nia.nih. gov/alzheimers/clinical-trials.*

A Word of Caution

Because Alzheimer's disease is so devastating, some people are tempted by untried or unproven "cures." Check with your doctor before trying pills or any other treatment or supplement that promises to prevent Alzheimer's. These "treatments" might be unsafe, a waste of money, or both. They might even interfere with other medical treatments that have been prescribed.

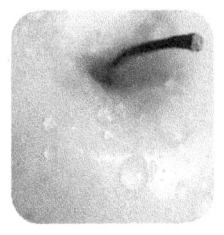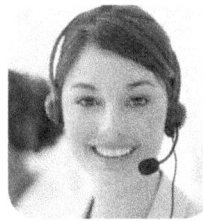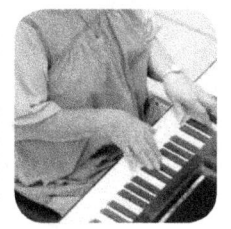

For More Information

Alzheimer's Disease Education and Referral (ADEAR) Center

P.O. Box 8250
Silver Spring, MD 20907-8250
1-800-438-4380 (toll-free)
www.nia.nih.gov/alzheimers

The NIA's ADEAR Center offers information and publications for families, caregivers, and professionals on diagnosis, treatment, patient care, caregiver needs, long-term care, education, training, and research related to Alzheimer's disease. Staff members answer telephone, email, and written requests and make referrals to local and national resources. Visit the ADEAR website to learn more about Alzheimer's and other dementias, find clinical trials, and sign up for email updates.

Alzheimer's Association

225 North Michigan Avenue, Floor 17
Chicago, IL 60601-7633
1-800-272-3900 (toll-free)
1-866-403-3073 (TDD/toll-free)
www.alz.org

The Alzheimer's Association is a national nonprofit organization with local chapters that provide education and support for people with Alzheimer's disease, their families, and caregivers. The Association also funds research on Alzheimer's.

Alzheimer's Disease Cooperative Study

University of California, San Diego
9500 Gilman Drive M/C 0949
La Jolla, CA 92093-0949
1-858-622-5880
www.adcs.org

The Alzheimer's Disease Cooperative Study (ADCS) is a consortium of NIA-supported medical research centers and clinics that develop and conduct Alzheimer's clinical trials.

Alzheimer's Foundation of America

322 8th Avenue, 7th Floor
New York, NY 10001
1-866-232-8484 (toll-free)
www.alzfdn.org

The Alzheimer's Foundation of America is a group of organizations that help individuals with Alzheimer's disease or other dementias. Services for consumers include a toll-free hotline that offers information and referrals, educational materials, conferences for caregivers, and a free quarterly magazine for caregivers.

ClinicalTrials.gov

www.clinicaltrials.gov

ClinicalTrials.gov is a registry of federally and privately supported clinical trials. Users can search for clinical trials and find information about each trial's purpose, who may participate, locations, and other details.

For more information about
Alzheimer's disease, please contact:

**Alzheimer's Disease Education and
Referral (ADEAR) Center**
www.nia.nih.gov/alzheimers
1-800-438-4380 (toll-free)
adear@nia.nih.gov

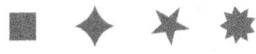

National Institute on Aging